I0455697

RENEWAL!

Renewal!

Techniques to Release Anxiety And Stress

Benita and Jim Babeckis

Published for:
TRANZFORMATIONS
Oro Valley, Az. 85704

Email: Tranzform@Comcast.net
Website: http:// Tranzformations.net

Published for Tranzformations
8571 N. Calle Tioga
Oro Valley, Arizona 85704

ISBN No. 978-1440413346

Copyright © 2007 by Benita and Jim Babeckis, All Rights Reserved.

All rights reserved. No part of this work may be reproduced or transmitted in any form by any means, electronic or mechanical, including photocopying and recording, or by any information s age or retrieval system, except as may be expressly permitted by the 1976 Copyright Act or by the publisher.

Type composition and design by Full Moon Rising.
Cover illustration by Jim Babeckis - Graphic Design and Illustration.
Copyright © 2007. Cover design by Full Moon Rising

If we have infringed upon any copyright material, we offer apologies, and we will give appropriate acknowledgments in all future editions once notified.

First Published October, 2008

Manufactured in the United States of America

Contents

Introduction

1. Why are We So Stressed ?

2. Block Behaviors That Keep Your Stress Alive

3. Stress or Anxiety?

4. Quiz Time!

5. Panic Attacks

6. Dealing with Panic Attacks

7. Calm Yourself with Visualization

8. Using Music to Beat Stress

9. Self-Hypnosis for Stress

10. Stress Management

11. More Stress Management

12. Who Ya Gonna Call? Stress Busters!

13. Just Say "No"!

Contents

14. Take a Break

15. Relaxing at Work

    Conclusions

Introduction

It seems like you hear it all the time from nearly every one you know – "I'm SO stressed out!" Pressures surround us in this world today. Those pressures cause stress and anxiety, and often we are ill-equipped to deal with those stressors that trigger anxiety and other feelings that can make us sick. Literally, sick. The statistics are staggering. One in every eight Americans age 18-54 suffers from an anxiety disorder. This totals over 19 million people. Research conducted by the National Institute of Mental Health has shown that anxiety disorders are the number one mental health problem among American women and are second only to alcohol and drug abuse by men. Women suffer from anxiety and stress almost twice as much as men.

Anxiety disorders are the most common mental illness in America, surpassing even depression in numbers. Anxiety is the most common mental health issue facing adults over 65 years of age. Anxiety disorders cost the U.S. $46.6 billion annually. Anxiety sufferers see an average of five doctors before being successfully diagnosed.

Unfortunately, stress and anxiety go hand in hand. In fact, one of the major symptoms of stress is anxiety. And stress accounts for 80 percent of all illnesses either directly or indirectly.

In fact, stress is more dangerous than we thought. You've probably heard that it can raise your blood pressure, increasing the likelihood of a stroke in the distant future, but recently a health insurance brochure claimed that 90 percent of visits to a primary care physician were stress-related disorders. Health Psychology magazine reports that chronic stress can interfere with the normal function of the body's immune system.

Studies have proven that stressed individuals have an increased vulnerability to catching an illness and are more susceptible to allergic, autoimmune, or cardiovascular diseases. Doctors agree that during chronic stress, the functions of the body that are nonessential to survival, such as the digestive and immune systems, shut down. "This is why people get sick," he says. "There are also many occurrences of psychosomatic illness, an illness with an emotional or psychological side to it." Furthermore, stress often prompts people to respond in unhealthy ways such as smoking, drinking alcohol, eating poorly, or becoming physically inactive. This damages the body in addition to the wear and tear of the stress itself.

Stress is a part of daily life. It's how we react to it that makes all the difference in maintaining our health and well being. Pressures occur throughout life and those pressures cause stress. You need to realize that you will never completely get rid of stress in your life, but you can learn coping techniques to turn that stress into a healthier situation.

Benita and I have learned, somewhat, how to cope with stress, although, we are always learning new techniques and mechanisms.

So what we've done in this book is taken some of our own experiences and combined them with advice from experts to give you tools that will help you in stressful situations. We've also outlined different ways you can face debilitating anxiety and panic attacks that many people suffer from.

While researching this book, we have come across some amazing information and can't wait to share it with you. We learned so much, so let's look at how to eliminate stress and anxiety from your life!

Chapter 1:

Why Are We So Stressed?

We're living in very trying and difficult times and things don't seem to be getting any easier. Sometimes life can seem terribly painful and unfair, yet somehow we manage to struggle on, day after day, hoping and praying that things will soon get better. But day by day the world is becoming a crazier and more uncertain place to live in, not to mention stressful. Nothing seems safe anymore. Millions of people are in record levels of debt. Many are losing their jobs, their homes, their health and sometimes even their sanity. Worry, depression and anxiety seem to have become a way of life for way too many people. We seem to have entered the Age of Anxiety. In fact, recently, the cover of Time magazine proclaimed this loud and clear on one of their covers as the featured story in that issue. The constant stress and uncertainties of living in the 21st century have certainly taken their toll, and as a result many of us seem to live a life of constant fear and worry.

When the terrorist attacks happened on September 11, this constant stress and worry seemed to just be magnified. In fact, many people even now four years later report they are still scared that something of that magnitude could happen again – perhaps closer to them.

Turn on the news or open up a newspaper and we are bombarded with disturbing images and stories. We begin to wonder if we are safe anywhere. In this, the information age, never before have we had so much access to so much data. The economy is another stressor. Our country is in debt and so are many Americans. Soaring gas prices, outrageous housing costs, even the cost of food has sent many Americans to work in jobs that are unsatisfying and tedious. They work these jobs because they need a paycheck. Today, it's more important to bring home the bacon rather than work in a dream career. Having more women in the workplace adds to the stress. So many women feel the need to be everything to everyone and that includes a paycheck earner, house keeper, mom, wife, daughter, and sibling. The only problem with that is some women just don't make any time for themselves thus contributing to their stress levels being at an all-time high. Even children can feel the pressure of stress and anxiety. Teenagers who want to go to college find themselves pushing themselves during their studies to try and obtain scholarships so they can attend schools that have ever increasing tuition costs. They find themselves having to hold down part-time jobs on top of all that to earn money for extras that their parents can no longer afford. Add peer pressure into the mix and you have a veritable pressure cooker! Cell phones, internet, palm pilots, blackberries, i-pods – we are always on the go and always reachable. We don't make time to relax and enjoy life any more. Why not? We certainly should! We feel pressure to do these things because we think we HAVE to, not because we WANT to. All too often, it's difficult for people to just say "No". Not saying that one little word piles up un-needed expectations and obligations that make us feel anxious.

All of us will experience situations that may cause us to become stressed or feel anxious. The reasons are too many to note but can include, buying a property, having guests stay over (in-laws!), being bullied, exams, looking after children, managing finances, relationship issues, traveling etc.

Stress is a 'normal' function of everyday life. Only when it appears to take over our lives does it then become a problem. Everyone will have different reasons why a situation causes them pressure. As a rule it's usually when we don't feel in control of a situation, then we feel its grip tightening around us causing us to feel worried or 'stressed'.

If stress is caused by us not feeling in control of a situation, the answer is to try and reverse this, and regain that control.

The good news is: YOU CAN! You have everything inside you that you need to overcome your stress and the accompanying anxiety. The problem is, often we don't realize that we are in control because we feel so out of control at time. But the tools are there, you just have to use them. Let's first look at the barriers we put up that are preventing us from becoming healthy and getting rid of our anxiety and stress.

Chapter 2:

Block Behaviors That Keep Your Stress Alive

There are three obsessive behaviors that you are likely to be engaging in that impede your healing process and stop you from enjoying a stress-free life. Recognizing these barriers can be a great first step toward getting rid of the problems that go with being too stressed.

The first is obsessive negativity. When you are obsessively negative, it means that you have a tendency toward being "negative" about people, places, situations, and things in your life. Perhaps you find yourself saying things like "I can't do this!" or "No one understands!" or "Nothing ever works!", for example. You may be doing this unconsciously, but essentially you have what's known as a "sour grapes" attitude, and it holds you back from knowing what it's like to view life from a positive lens and enjoy the beauty in yourself and people around you! There's a whole world out there for you with happiness and positive thinking.

Then you have obsessive perfectionism.

When you engage in obsessive perfectionism, you are centered on trying to do everything "just so" to the point of driving yourself into an anxious state of being. You may find yourself making statements such as, "I have to do this right, or I'll be a failure!" or "If I am not precise, people will be mad at me!" Again, this behavior may be totally under the threshold of your awareness, but it interferes greatly with your ability to enjoy things without feeling "uptight" and "stressed." Finally there is obsessive analysis. When you are obsessed about analyzing things, you find yourself wanting to re-hash a task or an issue over and over again. For instance, you might find yourself making statements such as, "I need to look this over, study it, and know it inside and out...or else I can't relax!" or "If I relax and let things go without looking them over repeatedly, things go wrong!" While analytical thinking is an excellent trait, if it's done in excess you never get to stop and smell the roses because you're too busy trying to analyze everything and everyone around you. Gaining insight into this type of behavior is one of the most important keys to letting go of stress, and getting complete power over your anxiety.

If you find yourself engaging in any of the above "Blocking Behaviors", there are two things you can do to help yourself.

First, ask the people you know, love, and trust, "Am I negative about things?", "Do I complain a lot?", and "Am I difficult to be around?" This may be hard for you to listen to, as the truth sometimes hurts a great deal. But the insight you will get from others' assessment of you is invaluable, and you'll know precisely how others see you. Accept their comments as helpful info, and know that you will gain amazing insights from what you hear.

Second, keep a journal to write down and establish patterns of when you are using "blocking behaviors." Even if you are not thrilled with the idea of writing, you can make little entries into a note book or journal each day. The great part is that you'll begin to see patterns in your behavior that reveal exactly what you're doing to prevent yourself from curing your anxiety. We'll give you some great stress busting techniques later in the book, but you need to recognize these blockages first so you can move into the "healing" stage and conquer your stress and anxiety. Many people think that stress and anxiety are the same thing. This couldn't be further from the truth!

Chapter 3:

Stress Or Anxiety

Contrary to popular belief, there is a difference between stress and anxiety. Stress comes from the pressures we feel in life, as we are pushed by work or any other task that puts undue pressure on our minds and body, adrenaline is released, extended stay of the hormone causes depression, a rise in the blood pressure and other negative changes and effects. One of these negative effects is anxiety. With anxiety, fear overcomes all emotions accompanied by worry and apprehension, making a person a recluse and a bagful of jitters. Other symptoms are chest pains, dizziness, and shortness of breath and panic attacks. Stress is caused by an existing stress-causing factor or stressor. Anxiety is stress that continues after that stressor is gone. Stress can come from any situation or thought that makes you feel frustrated, angry, nervous, or even anxious. What is stressful to one person is not necessarily stressful to another.

Anxiety is a feeling of apprehension or fear and is almost always accompanied by feelings of impending doom. The source of this uneasiness is not always known or recognized, which can add to the distress you feel.

Stress is the way our bodies and minds react to something which upsets our normal balance in life; an example of stress is the response we feel when we are frightened or threatened. During stressful events our adrenal glands release adrenaline, a hormone which activates our body's defense mechanisms causing our hearts to pound, blood pressure to rise, muscles to tense, and the pupils of our eyes to dilate. A principal indication of increased stress is an escalation in your pulse rate; however, a normal pulse rate doesn't necessarily mean you aren't stressed. Constant aches and pains, palpitations, anxiety, chronic fatigue, crying, over or under- eating, frequent infections, and a decrease in your sexual desire are signs you may notice which indicate you may be under stress. Of course, every time we are under stress, we do not react to such an extreme and we are not always under such great duress or fear every time we are confronted with a stressful situation. Some people are more susceptible than others to stress; for some, even ordinary daily decisions seem insurmountable. Deciding what to have for dinner or what to buy at the store, is a seemingly,monumental dilemma for them. On the other hand, there are those people, who seem to thrive under stress by becoming highly productive being driven by the force of pressure. Research shows women with children have higher levels of stress related hormones in their blood than women without children. Does this mean women without children don't experience stress? Absolutely not! It means that women without children may not experience stress as often or to the same degree which women with children do. This means for women with children, it's particularly important to schedule time for yourself; you will be in a better frame of mind to help your children and meet the daily challenge of being a parent, once your stress level is reduced.

Anxiety, on the other hand, is a feeling of unease. Everybody experiences it when faced with a stressful situation, for example before an exam or an interview, or during a worrying time such as illness. It is normal to feel anxious when facing something difficult or dangerous and mild anxiety can be a positive and useful experience. However, for many people, anxiety interferes with normal life. Excessive anxiety is often associated with other psychiatric conditions, such as depression. Anxiety is considered abnormal when it is very prolonged or severe, it happens in the absence of a stressful event, or it is interfering with everyday activities such as going to work. The physical symptoms of anxiety are caused by the brain sending messages to parts of the body to prepare for the "fight hormones,or flight" response. The heart, lungs and other parts of the body work faster. The brain also releases stress including adrenaline. Common indicators of excessive anxiety include:

- Diarrhea
- Dry mouth
- Rapid heartbeat or palpitations
- Insomnia
- Irritability or anger
- Inability to concentrate
- Fear of being "crazy"

Feeling unreal and not in control of your actions which is called depersonalization

Anxiety can be brought on in many ways. Obviously, the presence of stress in your life can make you have anxious thoughts. Many people who suffer from anxiety disorders occupy their minds with excessive worry. This can be worry about anything from health matters to job problems to world issues.

Certain drugs, both recreational and medicinal, can also lead to symptoms of anxiety due to either side effects or withdrawal from the drug. Such drugs include caffeine, alcohol, nicotine, cold remedies, and decongestants, bronchodilators for asthma, tricyclic antidepressants, cocaine, amphetamines, diet pills, ADHD medications, and thyroid medications.

A poor diet can also contribute to stress or anxiety for example, low levels of vitamin B12. Performance anxiety is related to specific situations, like taking a test or making a presentation in public.

Post traumatic stress disorder (PTSD) is a stress disorder that develops after a traumatic event like war, physical or sexual assault, or a natural disaster. In very rare cases, a tumor of the adrenal gland (pheochromocytoma) may be the cause of anxiety.

This happens because of an overproduction of hormones responsible for the feelings and symptoms of anxiety. While anxiety may seem a bit scary, what's even scarier is that excessive anxiety and stress can lead to depression. Suffering from depression can be a lifelong struggle as I well know, but the good news is that all of this is manageable! So, let's take a few little quizzes to see if you are suffering from too much stress, excessive anxiety, or depression.

Chapter 4:

QUIZ TIME!

Before you begin here, let us tell you that we are not medical professionals. This information has come from reliable sources and isn't meant to be a complete diagnostic tool in any way. These quizzes are simply guidelines to help you recognize any problems you might have and be able to effectively deal with those problems. Because depression can be the most serious of our topics, let's start by seeing if you may be depressed. Keep in mind that everyone has their "blue" days. The thing that separates clinical depression from simple melancholy is that the symptoms occur over a period of time. They don't come and go, they stay around for awhile and can affect your life adversely. Ask yourself the following questions. Answer yes if you've been feeling this way consistently over a period of two weeks.

1. Do you find yourself constantly sad?
2. Are you unmotivated to do simple things like shower, clean up the house, or make dinner?
3. Do people tell you you're overly irritable?
4. Do you have trouble concentrating?
5. Are you feeling isolated from family and friends even when they are around you?
6. Have you lost interest in your favorite activities?
7. Do you feel hopeless, worthless, or guilty for no reason at all?
8. Are you always tired and have trouble sleeping?
9. Has your weight fluctuated significantly?

If you can answer "Yes" to five or more of these questions, you could be suffering from clinical depression. It is important for you to seek out the help of a medical professional whether that be a doctor or a therapist. There are many medications out there that can help with depression.

As a friend of ours observed "We always try to deny our own depression, but once you began taking an anti-depressant, you can't believe what a difference that one pill a day will make! It gave me freedom from the "black hole" I had fallen into and helped me enjoy life again." So if you think you are depressed, ACT NOW! You deserve to be happy!

But this book is about stress and anxiety, so let's see if you are overly stressed. Ask yourself the following:

1. Do you worry constantly and cycle with negative self-talk?

2. Do you have difficulty concentrating?

3. Do you get mad and react easily?

4. Do you have recurring neck or headaches?

5. Do you grind your teeth?

6. Do you frequently feel overwhelmed, anxious or depressed?

7. Do you feed your stress with unhealthy habits eating or drinking excessively, smoking, arguing, or avoiding yourself and life in other ways?

8. Do small pleasures fail to satisfy you?

9. Do you experience flashes of anger over a minor problem?

If you can answer "Yes" to most of these questions, then you do have excessive stress in your life. The good news is that you've bought this book and will learn many valuable techniques to cope with that stress.

Let's move on to anxiety.

1. Do you experience shortness of breath,
    heart palpitation or shaking while at rest?
2. Do you have a fear of losing control or
    going crazy?
3. Do you avoid social situations because of fear?
4. Do you have fears of specific objects?
5. Do you fear that you will be in a place or
    situation from which you cannot escape?
6. Do you feel afraid of leaving your home?
7. Do you have recurrent thoughts or
    images that refuse to go away?
8. Do you feel compelled to perform
    certain activities repeatedly?
9. Do you persistently relive an upsetting
    event from the past?

Answering "Yes" to more than four of these questions can indicate an anxiety disorder. Suffering from depression, too much stress, or excessive anxiety can endanger your overall health and it's time to take steps to overcome this – RIGHT NOW!

Stress and anxiety affects many factors in our body not only in our mental state. Cancer and other deadly diseases are related to stress and anxiety because of the changes in the chemical composition in our body due to stress and anxiety.

You don't have to be a victim of stress and anxiety, its just all about discipline and having a proper schedule. Not taking in anything you cannot handle will be a lot of help. Learn your limitations and stick to it. Do not over exert yourself. Just try to go over the border an inch at a time. You can lead a productive successful and fulfilling life and career without the need to endanger your health. If not, you are not only killing yourself, you are also sending your family and friends and all the people around you away. Stress is a natural part of life. It can be both physical and mental and much of it can come from everyday pressures. Everyone handles stress differently, some better than others.

Left unchecked, however, stress can cause physical, emotional, and behavioral disorders which can affect your health, vitality, and peace-of-mind, as well as personal and professional relationships. As we've said, stress and anxiety can lead to panic attacks. Speaking from experience, I can tell you that having a panic attack can be a serious situation. Let's explore that subject a little more.

Chapter 5:

Panic Attacks

One of the unfortunate outcomes from suffering from excessive stress and anxiety is the physical reaction of your body to the situation. It's like your body is telling you that you need to rest for a moment. Except when you're having a panic attack, it's anything BUT restful. A friend of ours relates: "I had my first panic attack while my husband and I were driving home from a St. Louis Rams football game. We were about 30 miles from our home when I began to feel a bit "off". I was having trouble breathing, my body felt disconnected, and my heart was beating at what seemed like 90 miles an hour. I pulled the van off to the side of the highway and got out hoping to "walk it off." But it didn't work. No matter what I tried, I couldn't catch my breath. I felt like I was dying. I remember saying over and over again, "Please not now. I'm not ready." It was horrifying. The good news is that I wasn't dying – obviously! But that night began a terrible journey for me into how my body reacted to excessive stress and anxiety. Since then, I have had many panic attacks, but I also learned how to recognize that one might be coming on and how to control it.

I'm not always able to get hold of it completely and will occasionally fall into full-blown panic mode, but it's a lot better than it was." So, let's look at the signs that you might be having a panic attack. The following list gives tell-tale warning signs of an oncoming panic attack.

- Palpitations.
- A pounding heart, or an accelerated heart rate.
- Sweating.
- Trembling or shaking.
- Shortness of breath.
- A choking sensation.
- Chest pain or discomfort.
- Nausea or stomach cramps.
- De-realization (a feeling of unreality)

- Fear of losing control or going crazy.
- Fear of dying.
- Numbness or a tingling sensation in your face and limbs.
- Chills or hot flashes.

You would be surprised at how many people go to the hospital emergency room completely sure that they're having a heart attack only to find out that it's a panic attack. They're that intense!

It's very difficult for your loved ones to imagine or even understand what you are going through when you have a panic attack. They may lose patience with you, tell you to "get over it", or think you're faking. It may help if you show them the following scenario.

You are standing in line at the grocery store. It's been a long wait but there's only one customer to go before you make it to the cashier. Wait, what was that?

An unpleasant feeling forms in your throat, your chest feels tighter, now a sudden shortness of breath, and what do you know—your heart skips a beat. "Please, God, not here." You make a quick scan of the territory —is it threatening? Four unfriendly faces are behind you and one person is in front. Pins and needles seem to prick you through your left arm, you feel slightly dizzy, and then the explosion of fear as you dread the worse. You are about to have a panic attack. There is no doubt in your mind now that this is going to be a big one. Okay, time for you to focus.

You know how to deal with this – at least you hope you do! Start breathing deeply - in through the nose, out through the mouth.

Think relaxing thoughts, and again, while breathing in, think "Relax," and then breathe out. But it doesn't seem to be having any positive effect; in fact, just concentrating on breathing is making you feel self-conscious and more uptight. Maybe if you just try to relax your muscles. Tense both shoulders, hold for 10 seconds, then release. Try it again. Nope, still no difference. The anxiety is getting worse and the very fact that you are out of coping techniques worsens your panic. If only you were surrounded by your family, or a close friend were beside you so you could feel more confident in dealing with this situation.

Now, the adrenaline is really pumping through your system, your body is tingling with uncomfortable sensations, and now the dreaded feeling of losing complete control engulfs your emotions. No one around you has any idea of the sheer terror you are experiencing. For them, it's just a regular day and another frustratingly slow line at the grocery store. You realize you are out of options. It's time to run.

You excuse yourself from the line looking embarrassed as it is now that it is your turn to pay. The cashier is looking bewildered as you leave your shopping behind and stroll towards the door.

There is no time for excuses—you need to be alone. You leave the supermarket and get into your car to ride it out alone. You wonder whether or not this one was the big one. The one you fear will push you over the edge mentally and physically. Ten minutes later the panic subsides. It's only 11:00 in the morning, how in the world can you make it through the rest of your day

If you suffer from panic or anxiety attacks, the above scenario probably sounds very familiar. It may have even induced feelings of anxiety and panic just reading it.

The particular situations that trigger your panic and anxiety may differ. Maybe the bodily sensations are a little different. What's important to realize is that panic attacks are very real to the people who are having them and they should never be pushed off to the side. I remember one evening at home when I was by myself watching one of my favorite television programs. I thought I was in a safe place. There was no obvious trigger and I felt completely relaxed. Out of nowhere, I began having symptoms of a panic attack. The four walls of my living room were closing in around me. I couldn't breathe and felt like I was dying. I stepped out on my front porch for some fresh air and began deep breathing exercises. The symptoms eventually went away, but it left me wondering why exactly I had that attack. There was no obvious reason, no stressful situation, and no indicator that a panic attack might be impending. That's the strange thing about panic. Sometimes your mind can play tricks on you. Even when you think you're in no danger of having a panic attack, your brain might be feeling differently. That's the scary part. The good part is that there are ways you can combat panic attacks and cope much better when you find yourself in that situation.

Chapter 6:

Dealing With Panic Attacks

If you have panic attacks, it may help to comfort you that you are not alone! You're not even one in a million. In America, it is estimated that almost 5% of the population suffer from some form of anxiety disorder. For some, it may be the infrequent panic attacks that only crop up in particular situations-like when having to speak in front of others, while, for other people, it can be so frequent and recurring that it inhibits them from leaving their home. Frequent panic attacks often develop into what medical physicians refer to as an anxiety disorder. There are many ways of coping with an anxiety disorder. Some may not work for you, but others just might. It helps to know some of the most common coping techniques for dealing with panic before they begin. Your first step is to recognize when a panic attack is about to begin. When you have enough of them, you start to really pay attention to the tingling sensation, the shortness of breath, and the disconnection from the real life around you. Many people we talk to wonder what that disconnection is like. They have a hard time understanding it. Those of us who have panic attacks are all too familiar with it. It's like you can look at a solid object and see that it is there. You know it's there, but a part of your mind doubts that it really IS there.

You may find yourself reaching out to touch that object just to be sure. You feel like you're not a part of the world around you. It's as if you are just a spectator in your own life with no control over anything around you. Believe us, this is a horrible feeling.

So how do you start trying to combat your panic attacks? What if I told you the trick to ending panic and anxiety attacks is to WANT to have one. That sounds strange, even contradictory, doesn't it? But the "wanting" really does help push it away. Does this mean that you should be able to bring on a panic attack at this very moment? Absolutely not! What it means is that when you are afraid of something – in this case, a panic attack – it will more than likely appear and wreak havoc. When you stand up to the attack, your chances of fending it off are much greater. If you resist a situation out of fear, the fear around that issue will persist. How do you stop resisting–you move directly into it, into the path of the anxiety, and by doing so it cannot persist. In essence what this means is that if you daily voluntarily seek to have a panic attack, you cannot have one. Try in this very moment to have a panic attack and I will guarantee you cannot. You may not realize it but you have always decided to panic. You make the choice by saying this is beyond my control whether it be consciously or sub-consciously

Another way to appreciate this is to imagine having a panic attack as like standing on a cliff's edge. The anxiety seemingly pushes you closer to falling over the edge. To be rid of the fear you must metaphorically jump. You must jump off the cliff edge and into the anxiety and fear and all the things that you fear most. How do you jump? You jump by wanting to have a panic attack. You go about your day asking for anxiety and panic attacks to appear.

Your real safety is the fact that a panic attack will never harm you. That is a medical fact. You are safe, the sensations are wild but no harm will come to you. Your heart is racing but no harm will come to you. The jump becomes nothing more than a two foot drop! It's perfectly safe. Anxiety causes an imbalance in your life whereby all of the mental worry creates a top-heavy sensation. All of your focus is moved from the center of your body to the head. Schools of meditation often like to demonstrate an example of this top-heavy imbalance by showing how easily the body can lose its sense of center. The key to overcoming panic attacks is to relax. That's easy to say but difficult to do. A good way to do this is to concentrate on your breathing making sure it is slow and steady.

One of the first signs of a panic attack is difficulty breathing, and you may find yourself panting to catch a breath. When you focus on making those breaths even, your heart rate will slow down and the panic will subside. Breathing more slowly and deeply has a calming effect. A good way to breathe easier is to let all the air out of your lungs. This forces your lungs to reach for a deeper breath next time. Continue to focus on your out-breath, letting all the air out of your lungs and soon you'll find your breathing is deeper and you feel calmer.

Ideally, you want to take the focus off the fact that you are having a panic attack. Try to press your feet, one at a time, into the ground. Feel how connected and rooted they are to the ground. An even better way is to lie down with your bottom near a wall. Place your feet against the wall (your knees are bent) and press your feet one at a time into the wall. If you can breathe in as you press your foot against the wall, and breathe out as you release it, it will be more effective. You should alternate between your feet. Do this for 10 - 15 minutes or until the panic subsides.

Use all of your senses to take full notice of what you see, hear, feel, and smell in your environment. This will help you to remain present. Panic is generally associated with remembering upsetting events from the past or anticipating something upsetting in the future. Anything that helps keep you focused in the present will be calming. Try holding a pet; looking around your room and noticing the colors, textures, and shapes; listening closely to the sounds you hear; call a friend; or smell the smells that are near you. Many people strongly advocate aromatherapy to deal with panic and anxiety. Lavender can have an especially calming and soothing effect when you smell it. You can find essential oil of lavender at many stores. Keep it handy and take a sniff when you start feeling anxious.

Try putting a few drops of lavender essence oil into some oil (olive or grape seed oil will do) and rub on your body. Keep a prepared mixture in a dark glass bottle for when you need it. You can even prepare several bottles, with a small one to carry with you. Other essential oils known to help panic and panic attacks are helichrysum, frankincense, and marjoram. Smell each of them, and use what smells best to you, or a combination of your favorite oils mixed in olive or grape seed oil.

You may want to prepare yourself BEFORE a panic attack happens. When you're not in a panicked state, make a list of the things that you're afraid will happen. Then write out calming things that tell you the opposite of your fears. Then you can repeat these things to yourself when the panic starts to come.

Prepare a list of things to do in case of panicked feelings, and it will be ready for you when you need it. Fill it with lots of soothing messages and ideas of calming things to do. We find this to be a very helpful tool and are never without our small notebook that has these positive affirmations in it. Panic can be a very scary thing to go through, especially if you're alone. Preparing for when the panic comes can really help reduce the panic, and even sometimes help to prevent it.

Another great tool to combating anxiety and stress is to use visualization.

Chapter 7:

Calm Yourself With Visualization

The purpose of visualization is to enable you to quickly clear mental stress, tension, and anxious thinking. The visualization can be used when feeling stressed and is particularly useful when your mind is racing with fearful, anxious thinking. This visualization process, when practiced frequently, is very effective for eliminating deep-seated mental anxieties or intrusive thoughts. To gain maximum benefit, the exercise must be carried out for longer then 10 minutes at a time, as anything shorter will not bring noticeable results.

There is no right or wrong way to carry out the visualization. Be intuitive with it and do not feel you are unable to carry it out if you feel you are not very good at seeing mental imagery. As long as your attention is on the exercise, you will gain benefit.

It is best to do this exercise in a quiet place where you won't be disturbed, and then when you are more practiced you will be able to get the same positive results in a busier environment such as the workplace. You should notice a calming effect on your state of mind along with a sensation of mental release and relaxation.

Either sitting or standing, close your eyes and move your attention to your breath. To become aware of your breathing, place one hand on your upper chest and one on your stomach. Take a breath and let your stomach swell forward as you breathe in and fall back gently as you breathe out. Take the same depth of breath each time and try to get a steady rhythm going.

Your hand on your chest should have little or no movement. Again, try to take the same depth of breath each time you breathe in. This is called Diaphragmatic Breathing.

When you feel comfortable with this technique, try to slow your breathing rate down by instituting a short pause after you have breathed out and before you breathe in again. Initially, it may feel as though you are not getting enough air in, but with regular practice this slower rate will soon start to feel comfortable.

It is often helpful to develop a cycle where you count to three when you breathe in, pause, and then count to three when you breathe out (or 2, or 4—whatever is comfortable for you). This will also help you focus on your breathing without any other thoughts coming into your mind.

If you are aware of other thoughts entering your mind, just let them go and bring your attention back to counting and breathing. Continue doing this for a few minutes. (If you practice this, you will begin to strengthen the Diaphragmatic Muscle, and it will start to work normally—leaving you with a nice relaxed feeling all the time.)

Now move your attention to your feet. Try to really feel your feet. See if you can feel each toe. Picture the base of your feet and visualize roots growing slowly out through your soles and down into the earth. The roots are growing with quickening pace and are reaching deep into the soil of the earth. You are now rooted firmly to the earth and feel stable like a large oak or redwood tree.

Stay with this feeling of grounded safety and security for a few moments. Once you have created a strong feeling or impression of being grounded like a tree, visualize a cloud of bright light forming way t past your toes.

above you. A bolt of lightning from the luminous cloud hits the crown of your head, and that ignites a band of bright white light descending slowly from your head all the way down your body, over your legs, and as the band of light passes over you, feel it clearing your mental state. It is illuminating your mind and clearing any disturbing or stressful thoughts that you may have been thinking about. Repeat this image four or five times until you feel a sense of clearing and release from any anxious thinking.

In finishing, see yourself standing under a large, luminescent waterfall. The water is radiant and bubbling with vitality and life. As you stand under the waterfall, you can feel the water run over every inch of your body, soothing you and instilling within you a sense of deep calm.

Try to taste the water. Open your mouth and let it run into your mouth, refreshing you. Hear it as it bounces off the ground around you. The water is life itself and it is washing away stress and worry from your mind and body. After a moment, open your eyes.

Try to use all of your senses when carrying out the visualization.

To make the pictures in your mind as real as possible, use your senses of touch, taste, and hearing. Feel the water trickle down your body; hear the sound it makes as it splashes over you.

The more realistic the imagined scenarios, the more benefit you will gain. Many people report very beneficial and soothing results from using these simple visualizations frequently.The mind is much like a muscle in that, in order to relax, it needs to regularly release what it is holding onto.

You can use any situation or location that will help calm you. We liken this to "finding your happy place". Maybe you feel relaxed in a swimming pool or on the beach. Imagine yourself there. Just make sure wherever you go in your mind is a place where you can be calm and rested.

By visualizing the different situations, you are allowing your mind to release. It is like sending a message to your brain that when you close your eyes and begin this process it is time for letting go of anything that it has been mentally holding onto, including anxious thinking.

In order to train your mind how to let go of the stress, it is important to practice this daily. With practice, you can learn to release all stress within minutes of starting the exercise. Your daily practice should take place before going to bed, as that will enable you to sleep more soundly.

Many people do not do these visualizations in the bedroom but some other room before going to bed.

That way, when they enter the bedroom and close the door, they are leaving the mental stress and anxious thinking behind them. Just be sure you have the opportunity to totally concentrate on your mentalimages.

Visualization as a tool for dealing with mental stress is very effective. If such visualization is carried out properly, you can reach a deep feeling of inner calm. This technique probably will not work in helping to end an anxiety attack, but it can help that attack from beginning. It is a very powerful support tool for ridding yourself of general anxiety sensations.

With practice, you find you go days without having anxious thinking interrupt your life, and importantly, this significantly reduces the level of general anxiety you feel. Visualization is simply a tool you can use to overcome anxious thoughts and feelings. Let's look at various ways that you can combat excessive stress – beginning with music.

Chapter 8:

Using Music To Beat Stress

Listening to music does wonder to alleviate stress. Everyone has different tastes in music. We should listen to the music that makes us feel comfortable. Sitting down and forcing yourself to listen to relaxation music that you don't like may create more stress, not alleviate it. Music is a significant mood-changer and reliever of stress, working on many levels at once.

The entire human energetic system is extremely influenced by sounds, the physical body and chakra centers respond specifically to certain tones and frequencies. Special consideration should be given to the positive effects of one actually playing or creating music themselves. Among the first stress-fighting changes that take place when we hear a tune is an increase in deep breathing. The body's production of serotonin also accelerates. Playing music in the background while we are working, seemingly unaware of the music itself, has been found to reduce the stress of the workplace. That's why so many retail places play music while you shop – to take your mind off the high prices! Music was found to reduce heart rates and to promote higher body temperature - an indication of the onset of relaxation. Combining music with relaxation therapy was more effective than doing relaxation therapy alone.

Many experts suggest that it is the rhythm of the music or the beat that has the calming effect on us although we may not be very conscious about it. They point out that when we were a baby in our mother's womb, we probably were influenced by the heart beat of our mother. We respond to the soothing music at later stages in life, perhaps associating it with the safe, relaxing, protective environment provided by our mother. Music can be one of the most soothing or nerve wracking experiences available. Choosing what will work for any individual is difficult, most will choose something they 'like' instead of what might be beneficial.

In doing extensive research on what any given piece of music produces in the physiological response system many unexpected things were found. Many of the so-called meditation and relaxation recordings actually produced adverse EEG patterns, just as bad as Hard

Rock and Heavy Metal. The surprising thing was many selections of Celtic, Native American as well as various music containing loud drums or flute were extremely soothing. The most profound finding was any music performed live and even at moderately loud volumes even if it was somewhat discordant had very a beneficial response. As we mentioned before, there is not a single music that is good for everyone. People have different tastes. It is important that you like the music being played. I recently picked up a rest and relaxation CD at Wal-Mart that has done wonders for me. It has the sounds of the ocean in the background while beautiful piano music plays. It's very soothing. One note here, it's probably not a good idea to play certain types of ballads or songs that remind you of a sad time in your life when you're trying to de-stress.

The reason is obvious. You're trying to relax and wash away the anxious thoughts. The last thing that you need is for a sad song to bring back memories you don't need anyway.

Here are some general guidelines to follow when using music to de-stress.

To wash away stress, try taking a 20-minute "sound bath." Put some relaxing music on your stereo, and then lie in a comfortable position on a couch or on the floor near the speakers. For a deeper experience, you can wear headphones to focus your attention and to avoid distraction.

Choose music with a slow rhythm - slower than the natural heart beat which is about 72 beats per minute. Music that has repeating or cyclical pattern is found to be effective in most people.

As the music plays, allow it to wash over you, rinsing off the stress from the day. Focus on your breathing, letting it deepen, slow and become regular. Concentrate on the silence between the notes in the music; this keeps you from analyzing the music and makes relaxation more complete.

If you need stimulation after a day of work, go for a faster music rather than slow calming music. Turn up the volume and DANCE! It doesn't matter if you can actually dance or not. Just move along with the music and do what feels good. You'll be shocked at the release you can feel!

When the going gets tough, go for a music you are familiar with - such as a childhood favorite or favorite oldies. Familiarity often breeds calmness.

Take walks with your favorite music playing on the walkman. Inhale and exhale in tune with the music. Let the music takes you. This is a great stress reliever by combining exercise (brisk walk), imagery and music.

Listening to the sounds of nature, such as ocean waves or the calm of a deep forest, can reduce stress.

Try taking a 15- to 20-minute walk if you're near the seashore or a quiet patch of woods. If not, you can buy tapes of these sounds in many music stores. This has been very calming for us – you should try it too!

There's another great relaxation technique that we have found in coping with anxiety problems: self-hypnosis.

Chapter 9:

Self-Hypnosis For Stress

A fellow author reports: "a few weeks ago, I was feeling particularly overwhelmed with stress and anxiety. It seemed like anything that could go wrong, did go wrong. I felt like I was spinning out of control. I happened to be writing a book on yoga and meditation at the time and came across a website that offered a downloadable mp3 hypnotic relaxation session. It cost me about $20 and it was the best $20 I have ever spent!"

There are plenty of places on the internet where you can get these downloadable sessions for a small fee. However, you can also practice self-hypnosis on your own. You first need to find a quiet place where you can fully relax and listen to your inner voice. You shouldn't try to make something happen. Let your mind listen and relax. A large part of achieving that hypnotic state is to allow it to happen naturally. Also, don't watch for certain signs or signals that you might be in a hypnotic state. We can guarantee that if you look for these signs, you won't be able to fully relax and gain the benefits that you would if you just let it happen.

There are lots of different ways to experience hypnosis. No two people will have exactly the same experience.

In one respect, though, everyone has the same experience: the hypnotic state is always pleasant! There are no "bad trips" in hypnosis. Keep in mind that self-hypnosis is a skill, and that you will continue to get better at it and, as you do, it becomes ever more powerful. It's a good idea to set up a schedule of practice, allowing yourself anywhere between 10 and 30 minutes, depending on how busy you are and how much time you have to spend at it. Practice during the best part of your day if you can and at a time when you are least likely to be disturbed by others.

Most people find it best to practice lying down, in a comfortable position, with as few distractions as possible. If you are bothered by noise while you practice you can try to mask out the noise with some other source of sound.

You can try stereo music in the background, or white noise if you like. If, like most people, you don't have a white noise generator, try tuning a radio receiver between stations. The static you get when you do that is similar to white noise. However this takes an older or cheaper FM receiver without a noise suppressor. Sometimes AM tuners can be used for this. This should just be in the background and not so loud as to be distracting.

The basic divisions of a hypnotic induction are relaxation, deepening, suggestion application, and termination.

1. Relaxation

Your first job in the hypnotic induction is to slow the juices down and get yourself relaxed. But don't try to force your mind to relax (whatever that means)! If you get yourself physically relaxed, your mind will follow. Relaxation – really deep relaxation – is an ability that most people have either lost or never developed. Some people can do it quite easily, though. They just let go of their tensions and let every part of their body become limp and relaxed. If you are one of these people, begin your self-hypnosis practice by getting nicely relaxed. Take your time. This is not something you want to rush. The time involved for the relaxation phase of your self-hypnosis induction can vary from half an hour to just a few seconds. It is an important part of the induction and should not be slighted. As you get better and your skill increases, you will recognize deeply relaxed states, and you will be able to achieve them in a surprisingly short time. But as a beginner, take your time. It will be time well spent.

A very popular method of deep relaxation is the Jacobson Progressive Relaxation Procedure. This involves tensing each of the major muscle groups of your body (foot and lower leg on each side, upper leg and hip, abdomen, etc.). Tense the muscle group for a few seconds, then let go.

2. Deepening Procedures

Once you have completed the relaxation phase of your self-hypnosis induction procedure, you can begin to deepen the relaxed state. At some time between the deep relaxation and the deepening procedures you will move into a hypnotic state. You probably won't know it, especially as a beginner, but it will happen sooner or later.

One of the first hurdles a beginner must get over is the compulsion to "watch for it." That is, you will keep waiting for hypnosis to happen, for some change in your awareness or the way you feel that will say to you, "You're hypnotized."

Watching for hypnosis will definitely get in your way if you don't get it out of your mind. Going into a hypnotic state is, in this respect, similar to going to sleep. If you try to catch yourself going to sleep – if you try to be aware of the precise instant in which you actually go to sleep – you are much less likely to go to sleep. "Watching" keeps you awake.

In this same way you will not know when you go into a hypnotic state (but that won't be because you lost consciousness – you won't). Later, after you have been practicing regularly for a few weeks or a month or two, you'll be much more familiar with yourself and how it feels to be hypnotized.

Does it take everyone weeks or even months to get into a good hypnotic state? Definitely not. Some people have an amazing experience the very first time they try it. Others might practice for several days, noticing nothing, then out of the blue they have one of those great induction sessions in which they know something stupendously good happened. But if you happen not to be one of these people, don't worry about it. Just keep practicing and you will eventually get there.

One of the most popular deepening procedures is the count-down technique. Hollywood also likes this one. That is why you see it in so many movies. That and the swinging watch.

To use the count-down technique you simply start counting downward from, say, 20 (or 100, or whatever). Adjust the countdown number to whatever feels right to you after you have practiced a few times.

Imagine that you are drifting deeper with each count. Other images and thoughts will probably intrude themselves as you count. That is natural. Just gently brush them aside, continuing with your counting.

The speed with which you count down should be natural; not too fast, not too slow. For most people this means counting at a rate of about one count for each two or three seconds. Do it at a rate that feels comfortable and relaxed to you. Some people like to tie the count with their breathing. As they drift deeper their breathing slows down, so their counting also slows down.

Don't count out loud, just think your way down the count. You want to avoid as much physical involvement and movement as possible.

3. Suggestion Application in self-hypnosis

Once you have reached the end of your deepening procedure you are ready to apply suggestions. What you have done during the relaxation and deepening procedures is increase your suggestibility. That is, you have opened up your subconscious mind at least a little bit to receive your suggestions. This works because of the particular, and peculiar, characteristics of the subconscious part of your mind.

The most common and easiest way to apply suggestions is to have them worked out ahead of time, properly prepared and worded, and memorized. It should not be too difficult to remember them because they should be rather short and you are the one who composed them. If you have them ready and remembered, you can simply think your way through them at this point.

Dialogue, or more properly monologue, is also okay. You just talk ("think" to keep your effort to a minimum) to yourself about what it is you want to do, be, become, whatever.

Don't say "you." You are thinking to yourself, so use the first person personal pronoun "I." Some suggestions can be succinctly stated in a somewhat more formal sort of way, like, "I am eating less and becoming more slender every day."

Elaborate suggestions are generally wordier and more of an ad lib: "Food is becoming less important to me every day and I am filling my time with more important and meaningful pursuits than eating. It is getting easier and easier to pass up desserts and other fattening foods . . ." and so on. Generally speaking, the most effective kind of suggestion is image suggestion. Image suggestions usually do not use language at all. You can liken this to seeing yourself in a calm, relaxed state while in the middle of a chaotic situation.

Actually see yourself in your mind's eye. Although people sometimes see immediate results from their suggestions, it is more likely to take a little time for them to kick in. So don't be impatient. On the other hand, if you have not begun to see some results within, say, a couple of weeks, you need to change your suggestions.

4. Termination

Once you have finished applying suggestions you are through with your induction and you can terminate your session. You could just open your eyes, get up and go about your business, but that is not a good idea.

You should always formally identify the end of every session. Doing this provides a clear boundary between the hypnotic state and your ordinary conscious awareness. A clear termination also prevents your self-hypnosis practice session from turning into a nap. If you want to take a nap, take a nap. But don't do it in a way that sleeping becomes associated with self-hypnosis practice. If you are practicing at bedtime and don't care if you go on to sleep, that is okay. But still draw the line in your mind to indicate the end of your self-hypnosis session.

To terminate the session, think to yourself that you are going to be fully awake and alert after you count up to, say, three. "One, I'm beginning to come out of it, moving toward a waking state. Two, I'm becoming more alert, getting ready to wake up. Three, I'm completely awake." Something like that. Self-hypnosis can work wonders when it is practiced on a regular basis. You'd be amazingly surprised at the level of relaxation you can get to. It's one of the best things I ever did for myself!

Now we should move on to stress management techniques in general. This could be a long chapter, but a very, very helpful one.

Chapter 10:

Stress Management

As we've said before, stress is a part of life. There's no getting away from it. In fact, some stress is good stress. You may not believe that, but sometimes stress can motivate us to do things we may not normally do in a relaxed state. Stress can make us brave enough to go forward when normally we might hesitate. We have to be resilient in order to effectively cope with stress and help it enhance our life instead of control it. How do you get strong and resilient? By learning how to take control of your stress and make it work FOR you instead of AGAINST you.

Recognizing stress symptoms can be a positive influence in that we're compelled to take action – and the sooner the better. It's not always easy to discern why you have the stress in each situation but some of the more common events that trigger those emotions are the death of a loved one, the birth of a child, a job promotion, or a new relationship. We experience stress as we readjust our lives. Your body is asking for your help when you feel these stress symptoms. We're going to give you many suggestions in this chapter. Not all of them will work for you, but we're willing to bet that some of them will.

There are three major approaches to manage stress. The first is the action-oriented approach. In this method, the problems that cause stress are identified and necessary changes are made for a stress free life.

The next approach is emotionally oriented and in it, the person overcomes stress by giving a different color to the experience that caused stress. The situation, which causes stress, is seen humorously or from a different angle.

We especially advocate this approach to stress management. Sometimes if you don't laugh at a situation, you'll cry – uncontrollably. That's no solution. So learn to see the humor instead of the doom.

The third way is acceptance-oriented approach. This approach focuses on surviving the stress caused due to some problem in the past.

The first stress management tip is to understand the root cause of your stress. No one understands your problem better than you do. A few minutes spent to recognize your true feelings can completely change the situation.

During this process, identify what triggered the stress. If someone close to your heart is nearby share it with the person. If you are overstressed and feel you are going to collapse, take a deep breath and count till ten. This pumps extra oxygen into your system and rejuvenates the entire body.

When under severe stress meditate for a moment and pull out of the current situation for a little while.

Stand up from your current position and walk. Stretch yourself. Soon you will find that the stress has lessened. This is because you have relaxed now and relaxation is the best medicine for stress. Smiling is yet another way of stress management. If you are at the work place, just stand up and smile at your colleague in the far corner. You will see a change in your mood. Learn some simple yoga or mediation techniques. You can also invent your own stress management tips. The basic idea is to identify the cause of stress and to pull out from it for a moment and then deal with it. Taking a short walk and looking at objects in nature is another stress reliever. Drinking a glass of water or playing small games are simple stress management techniques. The whole idea is change the focus of attention and when you return to the problem, it does not look as monstrous as you felt before.

Here are five quick steps you can take toward relieving stress:

1. Don't just sit there. Move! According to many psychologists, motion creates emotion. You might notice that when you are idle, it's easier to become depressed. Your heart rate slows down, less oxygen travels to your brain, and you are slumped somewhere in a chair blocking air from reaching your lungs. We challenge you right now, regardless of how you are feeling, to get up and walk around at a fast tempo. Maybe you might want to go to an empty room and jump up and down a little bit. It may sound silly but the results speak for themselves. Try it now for a few minutes. It works like magic.

Exercise can be a great stress buster. People with anxiety disorders might worry that aerobic exercise could bring on a panic attack. After all, when you exercise, your heart rate goes up, you begin to sweat, and your breathing becomes heavier.

Don't panic – it's not an attack! Tell yourself this over and over while you're exercising. Realize that there's a big difference between the physical side of exercise and what happens when you exercise.

2. Smell the roses. How do you smell the roses? How about investing some money to go on that one trip you've been dreaming about? Visit a country with lots of exotic places to jolt your imagination and spur your creativity. You need to detach from your daily activities and venture a little bit.

3. Help others cope with their problems. It is very therapeutic when you engross yourself in helping others. You will be surprised how many people's problems are worse than those you may be facing. You can offer others assistance in countless ways. Don't curl up in your bed and let depression and stress take hold of you.

Get out and help somebody. But be careful. Don't get caught up in other people's problems in an attempt to forget about your own. We are constantly being called by friends and family when they need to vent or get advice. There are times that we find ourselves worrying about those who call us and we get caught up in what they're going through. This just gives us more stress than we already have and we find that we have to step away and re-assess the situation and our priorities.

We're now to the point where we can tell them that we just can't deal with it right now and to call back later. Sometimes, they get upset, but more often than not, they understand. But B and I have learned not to get too upset about their reactions. If it won't matter in a week, it shouldn't matter right now.

4. Laugh a little. By now you've heard that laughter is a good internal medicine. It relieves tension and loosens the muscles. It causes blood to flow to the heart and brain. More importantly, laughter releases a chemical that rids the body of pains. Every day, researchers discover new benefits of laughter. Let me ask you this question: "Can you use a good dose of belly-shaking laughter every now and then?" Of course you can. What you are waiting for? Go a comedy club or rent some funny movies.

5. Wear your knees out. If there were one sustainable remedy we could offer you when the going gets tough, it would be prayer. Many people, depending on their faith, might call it meditation. It doesn't matter to us what you call it, as long as you do it.

There you have a few quick fixes when you're feeling stressed. Want more? No problem!

Chapter 11:

More Stress Management

6. Make stress your friend

Acknowledge that stress is good and make stress your friend! Based on the body's natural "fight or flight" response that burst of energy will enhance your performance at the right moment. I've yet to see a top sportsman totally relaxed before a big competition. Use stress wisely to push yourself that little bit harder when it counts most.

7. Stress is contagious

What we mean by this is that negative people can be a huge stressor. Negativity breeds stress and some people know how to do nothing but complain. Now you can look at this in one of two ways. First, they see you as a positive, upbeat person and hope that you can bring them back "up". If that's not it, then they're just a negative person and can't feel better about themselves unless those around them are negative as well. Don't get caught up in their downing behavior. Recognize that these kinds of people have their own stress and then limit your contact with them.

You can try to play stress doctor and teach them how to better manage their stress, but be aware that this may contribute more to your own stress, so tread lightly.

8. Copy good stress managers

When people around you are losing their head, who keeps calm? What are they doing differently? What is their attitude? What language do they use? Are they trained and experienced? Figure it out from afar or sit them down for a chat. Learn from the best stress managers and copy what they do.

9. Use heavy breathing.

You can trick your body into relaxing by using heavy breathing. Breathe in slowly for a count of 7 then breathe out for a count of 11. Repeat the 7-11 breathing until your heart rate slows down, your sweaty palms dry off and things start to feel more normal.

10. Stop stress thought trains

It is possible to tangle yourself up in a stress knot all by yourself. You start by saying to yourself: "If this happens, then that might happen and then we're all up the creek!" Most of these things never happen, so why waste all that energy worrying needlessly? Give stress thought-trains the red light and stop them in their tracks. Okay so it might go wrong – how likely is that and what can you do to prevent it?

11. Know your stress hot spots and trigger points

Presentations, interviews, meetings, giving difficult feedback, tight deadlines……. Our heart rate is going up just writing these down! Make your own list of stress trigger points or hot spots. Be specific.

Is it only presentations to a certain audience that get you worked up? Does one project cause more stress than another? Did you drink too much coffee? Knowing what causes your stress is powerful information, as you can take action to make it less stressful. Do you need to learn some new skills? Do you need extra resources? Do you need to switch to de-caffeinated coffee?

12. Eat, drink, sleep and be merry!

Lack of sleep, poor diet and no exercise wreaks havoc on our body and mind. Kind of obvious, but worth mentioning as it's often ignored as a stress management technique. Listen to your mother and don't burn the candle at both ends!

Avoid using artificial means to dealing with your stress. That means don't automatically pour a glass of wine when you think you're getting stressed out and don't light up a cigarette. In actuality, alcohol, nicotine, caffeine, and drugs can make the problem worse. A better idea is to practice the relaxation techniques we've given you. Then, once you're relaxed, you can have that glass of wine if you want.

13. Go outside and enjoy Mother Nature.

A little sunshine and activity can have amazing ramifications on your stress level and will enhance your entire outlook towards life. Your improved attitude will have a positive effect on everyone in your family and/ or circle of friends; things which seem overwhelming will soon become trivial matters, causing you to wonder what the predicament was. Not only will you be less stressed, you will be healthier, happier, and more energetic; ready to face whatever obstacles come your way.

14. Give yourself permission to be a 'kid' again.

What did you enjoy when you were a child? Draw; paint; be creative. Play with Play- dough, dance, or read. Play music, allow yourself freedom to express yourself without worry that you're not keeping with the image of who you are 'supposed' to be. Just relax and enjoy yourself.

We all have a little child in us and it's a good idea to allow expression of the child within from time to time. If we might say so, this suggestion is excellent and very therapeutic. We speak from experience. We can tell you that there is nothing more satisfying than buying a brand new box of 64 Crayons – the one with the sharpener in the box – and coloring away in a coloring book. Our grandson loves it when we use this stress buster!

15. Don't set unrealistic for goals for yourself.

Many of us set ourselves up for defeat simply by setting unrealistic goals for ourselves. For example, if you are dieting, realize you cannot lose 40 pounds in one or two months. Or maybe you are trying to reach a goal of obtaining a particular job position; whatever your goal is allow sufficient time to reach your goals and realize occasional setbacks may occur. If you reach your goal without any delays, you will be even happier with yourself for arriving quicker than you planned, but don't expect it. In fact don't expect anything; expectations and reality are often two entirely different things.

16. Learn it is OK to say 'no' occasionally.

Often, many of us feel we have to say 'yes' to everyone, every time we are asked for help and feel that we must respond in a positive fashion. But, remember, you cannot be all things to all people. You must first meet your own needs before you can truly give others what they need while at the same time keeping yourself happy.

17. You do not have to do everything your family, friends, and others ask.

Of course you can help others, but first make sure you have done what is necessary to take care of yourself.

18. Make time for yourself, your number one priority.

Once your own needs are met you will find you have more time for others. And you may find more pleasure in helping others when you don't feel that you must always put others needs before your own. We're not done yet! There are so many great ways to combat stress and anxiety. You deserve to get all the information you can. After all, that's really why you're reading this book, isn't it? Here's some more stress busters.

Chapter 12:

Who Ya Gonna Call? Stress Busters!

We really love this one and have used it many times ourselves!

19. Yell!

That's right, scream at the top of your lungs as loud as you can. While this may not be feasible in your home, it works great when you're in your car with the windows rolled up. Let out a guttural yell from deep down inside. It's liberating!

20. Sing.

As we said in the previous chapter, music can be extremely beneficial when getting rid of stress. Think how much better you can feel when you belt out "Copacabana" at the top of your lungs! Who cares if you can't carry a tune? You're doing this for you!

21. Take up a hobby like knitting or crocheting.

Don't worry about being good at it. It's the process that's beneficial. Sitting still while performing repetitive movements is calming and stabilizing for many people. It can be time to collect your thoughts.

22. Start a garden.

Even apartment-dwellers can do this. Inside in pots, pots on the patio, pots, a small spot in your yard. There is a little work to setting it up. Tending plants, fruits, vegetables, flowers and watching them grow, bloom, or yield food is rewarding. Avid gardeners say working a garden is the best way to control stress and worry. An added benefit is the creation of a more beautiful, restful environment.

23. Play with a dog or cat.

Experts say pet owners have longer lives and fewer stress symptoms that non-pet owners. Playing with your pet provide good vibrations – for you and for the pet! It's a form of social interaction with no pressure to meet anyone's expectations!

24. Look at the stars and the moon.

It can be a very humbling experience to lay on a blanket with your hands behind your head and gaze up into the night sky. It's more than humbling; it's downright beautiful and relaxing! Just the other night, my grandson and I got a blanket out and lay in the yard looking at the moon going behind the clouds and gazing at the stars. He's only three, so it's a fascinating experience for him, but looking at the sky through his eyes made it even more fascinating for me. I could feel all my worries melting away as we chatted about the astronauts that get to see the stars close up and how big the universe is while we remain so small. When you look at the vastness of the sky, you realize that our problems are small compared to the vastness of the universe. We also get great comfort from seeing that one bright star in the sky that is always above our house.

When B's best friend's mother died, we got out of the car after coming from her visitation and our friend's five-year old and I stopped to star gaze. She pointed out one particular star and said "That's my grandma. She's our guardian angel now." Every time I see that star, I know grandma's there and she'll help get me through anything!

25. Treat yourself to some comfort food.

But be careful or over-eating could become your big stressor. Enjoy in moderation and make yourself feel better. I love mashed potatoes and gravy and macaroni and cheese. Those are my comfort foods. But I make sure that I don't overdo it. I give myself just enough to bring on that calming feeling.

26. Swing.

Remember the feeling of sitting inside that little piece of leather on the playground as you sway back and forth and feel the wind whipping through you hair? Do that! If you don't have a swing in your yard, go to a playground and remember to pump your legs back and forth to see how high you can go. It's liberating!

27. Take a candle lit bubble bath.

Even you guys out there can benefit from a warm bath bathed in the soft glow of candlelight. Lay your head back, feel the bubbles and the warm water, and let your stress go right down the drain when you pull the plug!

Phew! There you have twenty-seven ways to relax and de-stress! You can come up with your own ways as well! The key, really, is to find something that makes you feel better when you are overwhelmed.

Chapter 13:

Just Say "No!"

One huge problem people who are overly stressed out have is the ability to say "No" when they need to. Maybe your mother wants you to take Grandma to the store, but you're in the middle of a big work project. Perhaps your best friend asks if you wouldn't mind babysitting her kids when you've already made plans to get a haircut. There's no reason why you have to say "Yes" to everyone. In fact, there are often many times when you should turn them down. If you find yourself agreeing to do things when you really don't want to, you're a people pleaser. In general, this isn't a bad trait to have, but it can be a huge stressor.

People pleasers think of other people's needs before their own. They worry about what other people want, think, or need, and spend a lot of time doing things for others. They rarely do things for themselves, and feel guilty when they do. It's hard being a people pleaser. People pleasers hold back from saying what they really think or from asking for what they want if they think someone will be upset with them for it. Yet they often spend time with people who don't consider their needs at all. In fact, people pleasers often feel driven to make insensitive or unhappy people feel better - even at the detriment to themselves.

Constantly trying to please other people is draining and many people pleasers feel anxious, worried, unhappy, and tired a lot of the time. They may not understand why no one does anything for them, when they do so much for others - but they often won't ask for what they need. This is the trap many fall into. One of our neighbors asked our advice saying: "I found myself always agreeing to do for others but when I needed those same people to help me out, they were always occupied."

A people pleaser may believe that if they ask someone for help and that person agrees, that person would be giving out of obligation, not because they really wanted to. The thinking goes - if they really wanted to help, they would have offered without my asking. This line of thinking happens because people pleasers themselves feel obliged to help and do not always do things because they want to. Sadly, people pleasers have been taught that their worth depends on doing things for other people. It's painful being a people pleaser – believe us, we know! People pleasers are not only very sensitive to other people's feelings, and often take things personally, but they also rarely focus on themselves. When they do take a moment for themselves, they feel selfish, indulgent, and guilty which is why they are often on the go, rushing to get things done. Because people pleasers accomplish so much and are easy to get along with, they are often the first to be asked to do things - they are vulnerable to be being taken advantage of. People pleasers were most likely raised in homes where their needs and feelings were not valued, respected, or considered important. They were often expected as children to respond to or to take care of other people's needs. Or they may have been silenced, neglected, or otherwise abused, thus learning that their feelings and needs were not important.

In many cultures, girls are raised to be people pleasers - to think of others' needs first, and to neglect their own. Many women have at least some degree of people pleasing in them. Men who identified with their mothers often do as well.

Since a people pleasers' focus is mostly on others and away from themselves. They often feel empty, or don't know how they feel, what they think, or what they want for themselves. But it's possible to change this pattern and to feel better about yourself. We managed to learn how to break out of this cycle. You can do the same thing if you see yourself in the above description. You want to know how? It's easier than you think!

First, practice saying "NO". This is a very important word! Say it as often as you can, just to hear the word come out of your mouth. Say it out loud when you are alone. Practice phrases with NO in them, such as, "No, I can't do that" or "No, I don't want to go there". Try it for simple things first, and then build your way up to harder situations.

Stop saying YES all the time. Try to pause or take a breath before responding to someone's request. You may want to answer requests with "I need to think about it first, I'll get back to you" or "Let me check my schedule and call you back". Use any phrase that you feel comfortable with that gives you time before you automatically respond with "YES."

Take small breaks, even if you feel guilty. You won't always feel guilty, but most likely in the beginning you will. Remember that your mental health is well worth the aggravation you may have to take from others. What's important is you. When you are healthy, those around you will be healthy!

Figure out what gives you pleasure. For example, you may like reading magazines, watching videos, going to a park, or listening to music. Give yourself permission to do those things and then enjoy them.

Ask someone to help you with something. I know this is a hard one but you can do it! After all, everyone else is asking YOU for favors, why shouldn't YOU ask THEM? Just be tolerant if they turn you down. Just because you have always told them "Yes" doesn't mean they always have to tell you "Yes".

Check in with how you feel and what you are thinking. It's important to be aware of these things; they're part of who you are. And then try saying what you feel and think more often. Just remember to have a little decorum in certain situations.

Many people pleasers believe that nobody will like them if they stop doing things for other people. If someone stops liking you because you don't do what they ask, then you're being used by them and probably don't want them as a friend anyway.

People will like you for who you are and not simply for what you do. You deserve to take time to yourself, to say NO, and to take care of yourself without feeling guilty. It's within your reach to change - one small step at a time! We think most people would be in complete agreement when we make this next statement.

McDonald's had it right – You Deserve A Break Today!

Chapter 14:

Take A Break

So often, we know inside ourselves that we need a break. That break might be a full-fledged vacation or a weekend getaway. Either way, getting out of the daily grind can be amazingly liberating and a huge way to get rid of stress and anxiety. Unfortunately, many people think they can't take the time to get away. This is toxic thinking. Get out and get away! How many times have you continued working, knowing that you are not giving 100% to the task at hand? How many times have you read or written the same sentence over and over again, as your mind keeps wandering and thinking about other things? How often have you wanted to take a break from the family or kids but feared the consequences of doing so? It's time for a break!

Why do we not allow ourselves the time to take a 'time out'? Perhaps we feel like we don't deserve it or that there's just too much to be done. There are many genuine reasons for needing to complete jobs and tasks; however we may also on occasion have 'hidden agendas' as to why we cannot stop for a break. Why?

In order to complete the job so quickly'. This type of person is often looking to impress others with their efforts, thereby increasing their ego in the process.

Maybe you think you just can't take the time off. "I can't stop; I just have to get this finished". Does this sound familiar? "I can't stop because the job has to be finished, WHY? So I can move straight on to the next thing, and the next, and the next etc..." This person will find that there is always something that has to be done, which will constantly prevent him/her from taking a break.

Maybe you just feel like you need to be needed. A mother managing the household, kids and other chores may feel as if her household will collapse if she were to put her feet up or take a weekend off! By not taking a break she can keep convincing herself that her role is crucial and the family would collapse without her input. This may indeed be true, but is still not a good enough reason to prevent her having a rest! Get rid of that thinking! You can get some amazing benefits just by taking a little time for yourself! Allowing your mind and/or body to rest can help re-focus your attention, sharpen your wits and increase motivation. In addition, taking time out helps to relieve stress, can aid the recovery of tired muscles and also promotes the discovery that there is more to life than just work.

Many athletes will tell you that an important part of their training routine is rest. Muscles need time to repair after a workout. Remember that your brain is a type of muscle as well. It needs time to rest and recuperate in order to perform at its best. By giving your brain time off, you'll be able to better concentrate and give tasks you once found difficult your full attention. They'll be easier, Really!

So you've decided that a break is in order. Good for you! A break can be anything from a 10-minute meditation session to a trip around the world, and anything in-between.

We feel that a break should be something that takes your mind off of a preoccupation with the everyday tedium of life. So depending on the time you wish to take towards relaxing you may enjoy reading, watching a movie, cooking, playing with the kids, riding a motorbike or driving, exercising or doing sports, traveling or simply sleeping. While you are taking this rest, above all, allow yourself the time to do it and don't feel guilty about. You will gain so very much by this time off, so enjoy the time you are giving yourself. Life will go on without you and contrary to what your mind might be telling you, everyone will survive – even when you're not there! Let everything go and concentrate on YOU just this once instead of everyone around you!

If you're feeling tired, unmotivated or just in need of a rest, don't be a martyr or look negatively at this. You may actually find that in reality, allowing yourself a break will actually help you ultimately become more efficient and effective in every part of your life. Plus you'll get the badly needed recharging of your "batteries" that you need and sorely deserve!

Work can probably be one of the most stressful places to be. You might think that none of these techniques can help you when you're around your co-workers. You couldn't be more wrong.

Chapter 15

Relaxing At Work

Coffee breaks aren't the only times when you can take a moment for yourself. Experience has actually taught Benita and I that coffee (or smoke) breaks can actually add to the stress you feel when you're at work. Some of the suggestions we've given you in this book can certainly be practiced at work, but, unfortunately, others cannot. Here's a tried and true method to help you relax at work.

First, find a place to sit. Sit up straight with your back against the backrest of your chair, your feet flat on the floor, and your hands resting lightly on your thighs. If possible, close your eyes. You may do the exercise without closing your eyes, but closing your eyes will help you relax a bit more. Do not clench your eyes shut. Let your eyelids fall naturally. Breathe in slowly through your nose, counting to 5. Hold the breath for a count of 5. Breathe out slowly, counting to five. Repeat.

This exercise is performed by tensing and holding a set of muscles for a count of 5, and then relaxing the set of muscles for a count of 5.

When you tense each muscle set, do it as hard as you can without hurting yourself. When you release the hold, be as relaxed as possible. Begin by tensing your feet. Do this by pulling your feet off the floor and your toes toward you while keeping your heels on the floor. Hold for a slow count of 5. Release the hold. Let your feet fall gently back. Feel the relaxation. Think about how it feels compared to when you tensed the muscles. Relax for a count of 5.

Next tense your thigh muscles as hard as you can. Hold for a count of 5. Relax the muscles and count to 5.

Tighten your abdominal muscles and hold for a count of 5. Relax the muscles for a count of 5. Be sure you are continuing to sit up straight.

Tense your arm and hand muscles by squeezing your hands into fists as hard as you can. Hold for a count of 5. Relax the muscles completely for a count of 5.

Tighten your upper back by pushing your shoulders

back as if you are trying to touch your shoulder blades together. Hold for a count of 5. Relax for a count of 5.

Tense your shoulders by raising them toward your ears as if shrugging and holding for a count of 5. Relax for a count of 5.

Tighten your neck first by gently moving your head back (as if looking at the ceiling) and holding for 5. Relax for 5. Then gently drop your head forward and hold for 5. Relax for a count of 5.

Tighten your face muscles. First open your mouth wide and hold for 5. Relax for 5. Then raise your eye brows up high and hold for 5. Relax for 5. Finally clench your eyes tightly shut and hold for 5. Relax (with eyes gently closed) for 5.

Finish the exercise with breathing. Breathe in slowly through your nose, counting to 5. Hold the breath for a count of 5. Breathe out slowly, counting to five. Repeat 4 times. And that's it! Perform this exercise whenever you need to relax, whether it's on a plane or in a car or anyplace else you may be sitting. Because this exercise may be very relaxing, it should not be performed while driving.

Over time, if performed regularly, this exercise will help you recognize tension in your body. You will be able to relax muscles at any time rather than performing the entire exercise. Perform at least twice a day for long-term results. You may develop your own longer relaxation exercise by adding more muscle groups. Pinpoint your own areas of tension then tense and relax these areas in the same way.

Maximize the relaxation benefits of this exercise by visualizing a peaceful scene at the end of the exercise.

See yourself on a warm, sunny beach, on a boat or any other place where you feel relaxed - in detail for at least 5 minutes. Remember the happy place? Go there and enjoy it!

Chapter 16:

Conclusions

If you've learned nothing from reading this book, we hope you realize and understand that there is NO WAY to completely eliminate stress from your life. What you can do is to learn how to make that stress work FOR you. Stress management isn't as difficult as it might actually seem. However, we can't emphasize this next point enough. If you think you have too much stress in your life, it may be helpful to talk with your doctor, spiritual advisor, or local mental health association. Because reactions to stress can be a factor in depression, anxiety and other disorders, they may suggest that you visit with a psychiatrist, psychologist, social worker, or other qualified counselor. We don't want to present ourselves as medical professionals. All we want to do is give you some tools to implement in your life to help you better cope with those things that make us overwhelmed and feel out of control. You may also want to look into time management tools in order to get rid of some of your stressors. When we feel like we don't have enough time to do the things that need to be done, that creates more stress and can lead to anxiety which, believe me, you don't want to have!

Stress management tips are simple cost effective methods to effectively check stress. They can be practiced anywhere and at anytime. Well, almost anywhere and anytime. If you feel you are in need of help, do not hesitate. You might not be correct always. The cause of your stress might be for no reason at all. But it might be physical in its roots. Someone else might be able to solve it easily. Understand your limitations and it can relieve stress to a large extent.

Stress is a normal part of life. In small quantities, stress is good—it can motivate you and help you be more productive. However, too much stress, or a strong response to stress, is harmful. It can set you up for general poor health as well as specific physical or psychological illnesses like infection, heart disease, or depression. Persistent and unrelenting stress often leads to anxiety and unhealthy behaviors like overeating and abuse of alcohol or drugs. Just like causes of stress differ from person to person, what relieves stress is not the same for everyone.

In general, however, making certain lifestyle changes as well as finding healthy, enjoyable ways to cope with stress helps most people. We hope that we have given you some great ways of dealing with the stress that we all feel.

Above all, remember that you are in no way alone in this battle. There are hundreds of thousands of people out there who feel overwhelmed and nearly completely out of control. That's why we wanted to give you this book. So you can find peace within yourself and realize that we're all on this big blue earth for a reason. You are too! Enjoy it and live life to its fullest. And when you feel yourself stressed or beset with a panic attack, relax, breathe through it, and know that there are many, many people who know exactly how you feel.

Remember Bobby McFarrin's philosophy and the song —

"Don't Worry, Be Happy!"

For Further Reading

1. The Relaxation & Stress Reduction Workbook (New Harbinger Self-Help Workbook) by Martha Davis, Elizabeth Robbins Eshelman, Matthew McKay, and Patrick Fanning (Paperback - May 3, 2008)

2. The Anxiety & Phobia Workbook, Fourth Edition by Edmund J. Bourne (Paperback - May 2005)

3. 100 Essential Steps to Less Stress and Anxiety by Angela Coldwell (Paperback - Mar 6, 2008)

4. Mindful Solutions for Stress, Anxiety, and Depression by PhD. Elisha Goldstein (Audio CD – Sep 27, 2007)

5. EMDR: The Breakthrough "Eye Movement" Therapy for Overcoming Anxiety, Stress, and Trauma by Francine Shapiro and Margot Silk Forrest (Kindle Edition - April 1998) - Kindle Book

6. Time Life Medical: Stress & Anxiety At Time of Diagnosis (VHS Tape – 1996) VHS:

7. Attacking Anxiety & Depression: A Self-Help, Self-Awareness Program for Stress, Anxiety & Depression by Midwest Center for Stress and Anxiety, Inc.

8. Anxiety & Stress Reduction by Eric Zeisler (Music Download) Download MP3 Song: $0.99

9. Stress, Anxiety, and Depression-Individual Use DVD Copy* (DVD – Dec 13, 2007)

10. The StressEraser Stress Reduction Machine by THE STRESSERASER

11. No Stress Passing - Humorous / Funny Long Sleeve T-Shirt by ArtApart

12. Heather (20 ml) (Calluna vulgaris) by Bach

Other Books by Benita and Jim

Benita and Jim Babeckis, *ABC's of Goal Setting.*

Ever set goals and write them down? What happened? Did you reach any of them or did you give up before you got there? Supercharge your goal setting and get ready for that satisfaction that only comes after reaching one of your goals. This book makes goal setting easy.

Benita and Jim Babeckis, *Life Management*

Are you organized? Then you aren't the person we're looking for. If you aren't as organized as you think you should be, this is the book for you. Say goodby to clutter and let order reign. We provide clever home and family management tips.; time saving tips and more. Get help managing your life.

Benita and Jim Babeckis, *You Want It When?*

Are you a procrastinator? Do you put off doing things until just before they're due? Do you do your Christmas shopping on Christmas Eve? There is help for all of you right here. Learn how to break the procrastination habit.

Put Your Weight Loss in Overdrive

Do you want to lose weight? Are you willing to eat healthier and make changes in your diet? If you are willing to follow our lead and replace your unhealthy diet with even some of the super foods we tell you about in this book, you will put your diet in overdrive. Weight loss will be a snap. ISBN # 978-1440413320

How Toxic Are You?

Everyone is subjected to toxins everyday. Over 80,000 at last count. Living away from the larger cities helps but not as much as you think. There are toxins in our water, our food, and in our air. What can we do to be healthy and survive our toxic world? Does fasting or jogging help? Yes, but not enough – toxins bind to fat cells. If you are at all interesting in your and your families health, this is a must read! ISBN # 978-140425590

An Introduction To Traditional Chinese Medicine

Tired of prescriptions? of taking hundreds of pills? You've probably wondered about acupuncture and chinese medicine but were afraid to take the plunge without knowing just a little bit more about what is involved and how it could benefit you. In *An Introduction To Traditional Chinese Medicine*, Benita and Jim will explain how Acupuncture, Yoga and Qigong can help you attain and stay healthy and what system of beliefs are behind how they work.
ISBN # 978-1440424586

Coming Soon!

You Were Born To Excel

This book is based on a series of classes we compiled back in June of 1998. The classes were called Human Excellence Engineering. The basic series consisted of six classes as presented in this book. Two to three weeks were spent on each class. An advanced series was planned and begun but never completed. The topics covered are: In chapter 1: New Thinking Skills; in chapter 2: Inside You; in chapter 3: Changing the Past; in chapter 4: A Brighter Today; in chapter 5: Feeling Good Again; and in chapter 6: The Future Begins Here. The classes and hence, the material in this book are a combination of NLP, Psychology and Shamanism. ISBN # (not yet assigned)

Personal Trance-formations

More than ever, researchers are concerned with the effects of mental and emotional states on an individual's health and with the possibility of treating the patient as an active and responsible participant in the healing process rather than as a passive recipient of either the disease or the cure. It is this emphasis that provides the basis for using a variety of techniques that enable non-medical persons to control pain perception and create their own response to illness. The mind plays a vital role in healing, more even than modern medicine has so far acknowledged. This guidebook to your inner world, the inner landscape of your soul, will help you connect with your most authentic feelings and thoughts. It contains a variety of techniques for dealing with this deep inner material. ISBN # (not yet assigned)

Approaching Wisdom

Storytelling is essential to the shaman's craft. There was more to the old tales than just a good yarn. Woven into the thrills and emotions were messages. The tales are the framework of the lore and the lore is a body of teachings and an essential part of the shaman's working life. Through lore we re- create the ancient strands of Otherworldly knowledge buried deep in our unconscious and bring them to the forefront of our conscious mind. We can then see them from a new perspective and apply them to life in our "everyday" world. This book recreates the shaman's storytelling as a quest for wisdom. In it we explore ways through story, myth and exercises to expand your sensory awareness, achieve internal union and contact your transpersonal self. This book provides tools, but the real exploration is up to you. ISBN # (not yet assigned)

The Castle of the Grail

The Quest for the Grail is not a fairy tale for children. It is a serious undertaking. The journey is full of trials and tribulations. The inner landscape of the Quest is full of dark forests, winding paths, narrow places, bridges, gates and castles. It is a very confusing place for us because we start foolish and ignorant. We do not recognize our guide and are frightened of what we might find. We are tested severely and ruthlessly but with mercy. The Quest is about Self Transformation and personal liberation. There is a unifying principle at the heart of all of these ways of thought, which can only be grasped by symbols, analogies and myths. Jung explained this with his archetypes of the collective unconscious. ISBN # (not yet assigned)

The Gold Mine in PLR.

What is PLR? How can it benefit you? P.L. and R. are the initial letters of Private Label Rights. PLR is merchandise or software, most of which is info or text based, customizable, and reusable as your own. The concept of PLR differs only slightly from having a ghostwriter. So if you have a website and need fresh content or are a writer and need fresh ideas - this book is a must have!   ISBN # (not yet assigned)

Creativity Workbook

Would you like to be more creative? More intuitive? Would you like to learn creative problem solving? You can with the proper training. You probably already are intuitive and creative without realizing it. This book will provide the training you need to handle anything life throws at you in a more creative way. ISBN # (not yet assigned)

Never Pay for Computer Software Again

Would you like to get a totally free operating system for your PC? How about an office suite that is rated better than Microsoft Office without Microsoft's price tag? Would you like free Image manipulation (Graphics) software? Games, Productivity software, Business applications - and all for free? How about one of the best web browsers around? Interested? It's all explained right here in Never Pay for Computer Software Again. Interested? You should be.
ISBN # (not yet assigned)

Surviving Life

How do you stay cheerful in the face of adversity, loss of job, bankruptcy, taxes and all the other things that life can throw at you?
ISBN # (not yet assigned)

Take Control (It's Your Book)

Covers everything the author needs to know about self publishing. Copyrights, ISBN numbers, writing software versus page layout software, cover design, book layout, POD versus conventional printing methods, marketing, distribution, advertising, etc. ISBN # (not yet assigned)

The Family Book of Fairy Tales

Stories of Princes and Princess's, enchanted giants and mighty ogres, lions, tailors and onions collected from around the world and assembled in this book to amuse you and your children. Includes the following stories: Cinderella's Daughter, The Giant's Hand, The Prince and the Lions, The Three Buns, The Boyer's Bride, How the Sea Became Salt, The Captive Princess, The Enchanted Oranges, The Knight of the Onion Shield, The Trade That No One Knew and The Prince and The Tailor. ISBN # (not yet assigned)

Benita's Encyclopedia of Crystals and Stones

What gems, crystals or stones have healing properties? Which do not? Which stones would you use for High Blood Pressure? Which for blood disorders? Which stones would be more effective for sores and wounds? How would you use Calcite in healing? ISBN # (not yet assigned)

Handy Order Form

Fax orders: 520-297-1293. (Send this form)

Telephone orders: 520-297-1293

(Have your credit card handy)

Email orders: Tranzform@Comcast.net <Attn. Orders>

Postal orders: Orders * 8571 N. Calle Tioga * Oro Valley, Az.

85704

Please send the following books, software or reports:
I understand that I may return any of them for a full refund for
any reason.

ISBN No. _____   Quantity ☐

Title: _____

ISBN No. _____   Quantity ☐

Title: _____

Name: _____

Address: _____

City: _____ State : _____ Zip: _____

Phone: _____ _____ _____

Email: _____

I would like more information on other books and/ or

products - ☐

Handy Order Form

Fax orders: 520-297-1293. (Send this form)

Telephone orders: 520-297-1293

(Have your credit card handy)

Email orders: Tranzform@Comcast.net <Attn. Orders>

Postal orders: Orders * 8571 N. Calle Tioga * Oro Valley, Az.

85704

Please send the following books, software or reports:
I understand that I may return any of them for a full refund for any reason.

ISBN No. _____ Quantity ☐

Title: _____

ISBN No. _____ Quantity ☐

Title: _____

Name: _____

Address: _____

City: _____ State : _____ Zip: _____

Phone: _____

Email: _____

I would like more information on other books and/ or

products _____ ☐

www.ingramcontent.com/pod-product-compliance
Lightning Source LLC
Chambersburg PA
CBHW060634290526
45793CB00001B/243